Nancy Rose Hunt

Suturing New Medical Histories of Africa

Carl Schlettwein Lectures

edited by the

Centre for African Studies Basel

Vol. 7

LIT

Nancy Rose Hunt

Suturing New Medical Histories of Africa

LIT

Cover image: Pharmacy at Yanonge, DRC
Nancy Rose Hunt, 2007

Text edited by Stephanie Bishop
Typesetting by Tilo Richter, www.trichter.de

Bibliographic information published by the Deutsche Nationalbibliothek
The Deutsche Nationalbibliothek lists this publication in the Deutsche Nationalbibliografie; detailed bibliographic data are available in the Internet at http://dnb.d-nb.de.

ISBN 978-3-643-90365-5

A catalogue record for this book is available from the British Library

Klosbachstr. 107
CH-8032 Zürich
Tel. +41 (0) 44-251 75 05
Fax +41 (0) 44-251 75 06
E-Mail: zuerich@lit-verlag.ch
http://www.lit-verlag.ch

LIT VERLAG Dr. W. Hopf
Berlin 2013
Fresnostr. 2
D-48159 Münster
Tel. +49 (0) 2 51-62 03 20
Fax +49 (0) 2 51-23 19 72
E-Mail: lit@lit-verlag.de
http://www.lit-verlag.de

Distribution:
In Germany: LIT Verlag Fresnostr. 2, D-48159 Münster
Tel. +49 (0) 2 51-620 32 22, Fax +49 (0) 2 51-922 60 99, E-mail: vertrieb@lit-verlag.de
In Austria: Medienlogistik Pichler-ÖBZ, e-mail: mlo@medien-logistik.at
In Switzerland: B + M Buch- und Medienvertrieb, e-mail: order@buch-medien.ch
In the UK: Global Book Marketing, e-mail: mo@centralbooks.com
In North America: International Specialized Book Services, e-mail: orders@isbs.com
e-books are available at www.litwebshop.de

FOREWORD

In September 2011 an international conference on the history of health care in Africa in the 20th century concluded a three and a half-year research project.* This bridged two of the five research axes at our Centre: Knowledge Production and Transfer on the one hand and Public Health and Social Life on the other. It brought together members of the history and anthropology departments of the University of Basel and drew support from the Swiss Tropical and Public Health Institute.

Close to 30 scholars – many of them leading historians in the field – from Africa, Western Europe and the United States presented their current research and discussed old and new findings in the history of health and medicine in Africa. The site for the conference, the monastery of Dornach, provided a suitable setting for the conclusion of the research project, which focused on the history of medical institutions founded by Swiss mission societies in Ghana, Tanzania and South Africa. The papers presented, however, went far beyond this empirical framework. The range of analytical perspectives chosen and of sources used by the participants reflected the diversity – the richness but also complexity – of the engagement with histories of health, healing, medicine, body, sickness and disease in general and in Sub-Sahara Africa in particular.

The Carl Schlettwein Lecture 2011 was presented on the first night of the conference by one of the most distinguished and innovative historians of health. Nancy Rose Hunt introduced a broad audience to the field of African Medical History and her lecture, at the same time, served as keynote address to the conference.

Nancy Rose Hunt is Professor of History (and Obstetrics/Gynaecology) at the University of Michigan, Ann Arbor. Educated in the humanities and especially medical history at the universities of Chicago (BA, 1980) and Wisconsin-Madison (PhD, 1992), she has taught and carried out research in Burundi, the Democratic Republic of Congo, and Ghana. *A Colonial Lexicon*, her widely received ethnographic history of medicine, childbearing, and therapeutic objects in colonial and post-colonial Zaire, earned the African Studies Association's Herskovits Prize in 2000.** Her new book, *A Nervous State: Violence, Remedies, and Reverie in Colonial Congo*, forthcoming from Duke, considers the sequelae of imperial violence on bodies, persons, communities, and states. Hunt is also busy writing Health & Medicine: A World History, a short primer with complex scales, for the new Oxford World History Series.

In a lecture that sutured a wide range of evidence into a lively narrative, Nancy Rose Hunt highlighted a range of advances in the history of health in Africa. The Carl Schlettwein Lecture linked the conference at the monastery in Dornach with the town of Basel and connected it with a broader public. It was a call on historians of health and medicine to reflect how we connect our work to the past, to the present, to the world and the local, to those who are concerned, and to those who should be concerned. The lecture made a deep impression on the audience and provided a great stimulus for the discussions at the conference. We are sure that Nancy Rose Hunt will inspire other colleagues to suture new medical histories in much the same way as she has inspired us.

Basel, 14 December 2012

Marcel Dreier, Patrick Harries, Brigit Obrist, Pascal Schmid, and Peter van Eeuwijk

* "The History of Health Care in Africa: Actors, Experiences, and Perspectives in the 20th Century," conference at the University of Basel, 12–14 September 2011.

** Nancy Rose Hunt, *A Colonial Lexicon: Of Birth Ritual, Medicalization, and Mobility in the Congo* (Durham: Duke University Press, 1999).

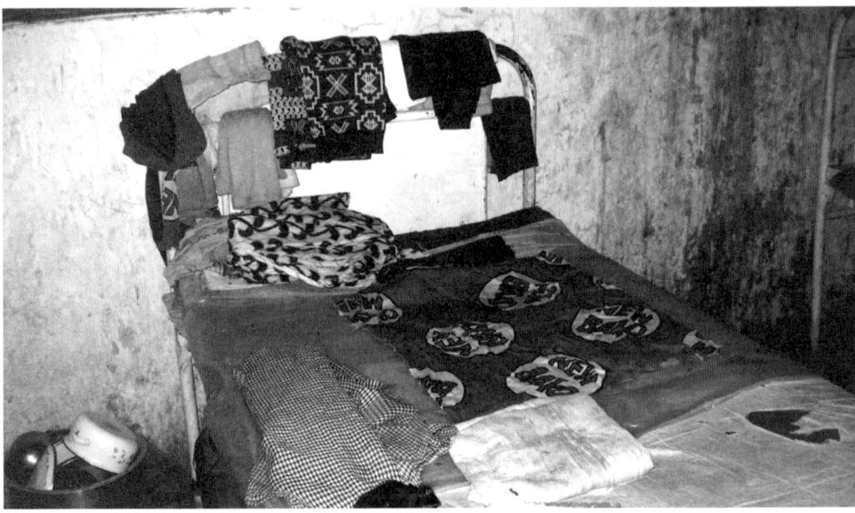

Bed at Yakusu Hospital, 2007 (N. R. Hunt).

SUTURING NEW MEDICAL HISTORIES OF AFRICA

I begin with a photograph, one of dozens I took during a trip in 2007 to former war zones in eastern Democratic Republic of Congo. This image of a patient's hospital bed comes from Yakusu, an old colonial mission hospital on the Upper Congo River. I snapped it not in 1989 when I first did research in the region, but in 2007 when this hospital founded in the 1920s was not exactly in ruins, but in serious disrepair with carcasses of surgical equipment laying around.[1] A hospital patient—or one of her family caretakers—covered her bed with pieces of cloth, creating a little homelike world of domesticity within this clinical ward about fifteen miles downriver from Kisangani. Most patients who come to Yakusu these days find old, rickety, metal bed frames when they move in for medical care. Some find a mattress available to set within the frame; surely some provide their own. This photograph gives one sense to contemporary hospital culture on this old British Baptist mission station, about a decade after the last missionaries from England and Scotland picked up and left due to insecurity and war.

What does this photograph have to do with my subject here, "suturing" and medical history? The patient (and kin) who occupied this bed pieced together odds and ends of available cloth. The result is a semblance of a bedspread, colorful, warm, likely comforting for some eyes and hearts. Whatever we might see within this image—

poverty or dignity or a quilt of near rags—it suggests modest means and a display of sorts about distinction, even pride.

Cloth as wealth is an old theme in African history. Hospitals, processes of making home, and domesticating spaces and persons also go together as an important theme in Africa's medical history. This carefully arranged hospital bed suggests much about paucity, survival, and making clinical space one's own. Each bit of cloth assembled across the bed or hanging from the bedstead probably contained its own story and value as a memory object in relation to past gifts, purchases, and special occasions. Together these cloth pieces suggest a certain calm, even poise and worth, although each separate patch of cloth seems to have been momentarily positioned rather than stitched into place.

2

I use this photograph to try to pry open some fresh thinking about medical history. My first question is: What kind of medical history is needed for Africa's present, for Africa today? My second hovers around issues of production, dissemination, and audiences. Who is producing African medical history, and *where*—in what kinds of intellectual, academic, public, corporate, and entrepreneurial locations? And who are we (scholars)—and others—producing it *for*? Clearly, the academy—from history and anthropology departments to tropical research institutes—values new work about the history of health, care, and biomedicine in Africa. At the same time, African medical history is situated in relation to new realities, quite unlike those of the 1970s when a small group of historians and anthropologists brought the African field of health, healing, and medicine to life.[2] We are now in a time of "global health," and we must reckon with this new creature and nomenclature head on.

Surely 9/11 and new security agendas have had much to do with the mushrooming of the new field and industry of "global health," once instead called "international health," an expression that worked quite well from about the 1920s. However we date and explain the emergence of global health, by 2003 a best-selling biography of Paul Farmer had appeared, global health publishing and funding had skyrocketed, and a new generation of health workers had found a hero in this remarkable story of a Harvard-trained, American medical doctor and anthropologist who set up clinics for the poor in Haiti, while railing against inequalities and structural violence and tackling significant global health problems.[3] Paul Farmer is an important face—and icon—of global health, and we can be grateful to him for the critical edge to his work and writing. Not all manifestations of global health in Africa are as inspired or laudable. But global health operations in Africa today—some more worthy, some more dubious—are the new *present* in relation to which most of us now write; and this fact alone has implications for how we conceptualize and cast our historical work.

3

So it is that I interject a new term and concept at this juncture of medical historical writing and thinking: suturing. It relates to the Yakusu patient's patchwork of a bedspread, and its meanings are many, some more complex, some mundane. The rich array is why I am drawn to this word that suggests, first and foremost, a surgeon busy at work, stitching, mending, with the aid of small manufactured technologies, sutures.

Of course, like all good scholars working in the English language, my exploration began with the *Oxford English Dictionary* (OED): A doctor joins the lips of a wound or the ends of a severed nerve with stitches, bringing the cut's edges together with a suture. A suture may also be an object, a device enabling this stitching work to hold. Anatomists, zoologists, and botanists speak of a suture as a juncture of two things—as in skull bones or shell parts—a junction that creates a line of closure, a seam joining and connecting two contiguous parts.[4]

Not all seams are straight, however, and just this recognition helps us think again of that *almost bedspread* in a patient ward of the aging, crumbling, still not abandoned Yakusu hospital. The bed covering consists of patches, scattered pieces of cloth with jagged edges, gaps, and holes. This patient's joining was temporary, perhaps even a daily hospital activity. The results suggest a semblance of a new abode made by self or a sister or mother. Some vanity and symbolic capital are lurking there in this photograph. Let's remember what most doctors, nurses, and medical anthropologists know about today's Africa—that most patients are somehow linked by cell phone connection to relatives near and far. Regardless, this patient managed to have the fanciest, if still humbly assembled, bed of cloth at Yakusu's hospital on the day I passed through in 2007.

The word suturing also has long had a literary connotation with, as the *OED* tells us, stitching carried into composition, as in "the seams" of a "literary suture." This kind of writing may involve extracting a passage from one text and resetting it in another, modifying some phrasing or punctuation in the process.[5] Historians often work like this, of course, cutting and pasting bits of primary source material into their writing. But let's not forget that suturing goes almost first and foremost with wounds; and, this emphasis is capital for an era when injury and trauma are ever more part of the vocabularies of historians working on colonial and postcolonial locations.[6] Indeed, my central question remains: If it is helpful to think of suturing as we go about producing our African medical histories, *why* is it helpful *now*?

Historians struggled with questions of narrative and emplotment in the 1980s. But textual metaphors have lost ground in our 21st century worlds, in good part because of the ways new media, digital, and communications technologies are marking and transforming all our lives, our ways of reading and knowing, telling and sharing, finding friends, voting, networking, and refusing.[7] Whether using cell phones or websites, social networking or scanning devices, from remote African villages to hyper-contemporary Basel, making and accessing knowledge has become more interactive and hyperlinked than ever before. And, more and more historians also work as creative co-engineers and co-designers in a brave, new, collaborative, academic world: the digital humanities.

The crucial reason I am drawn to the term suturing relates to the word's use and meanings in the worlds of media, cinema, and film. In film theory, suturing hails from a psychoanalytic lexicon about split subjects, subject positioning, and identification. It involves the way film is edited and cut to position viewers—spectators—to identify *or not identify* with characters, situations, and emotions. Some film theorists speak of suturing together the symbolic and the imaginary, that is, linking the linguistic (or word- and sign-based) with the visceral or emotional. Such junctions (often of two scenes or filmic bits) are designed to elicit in the film viewer a sense of the uncanny, a feeling that something scary is lurking though withheld. This kind of suturing in disrupts preferred readings and identifications through unsettling spectators, through producing disquiet within them.[8] Something analogous is apt for today's historians working among prose, images, and the digital.

Consider first a concrete example: a film about health and humanitarianism in Africa that *sutures*, and brilliantly so. It is a film I use to disconcert and provoke reflexive thinking when I teach African medical history and anthropology in North America to undergraduate students, most keen to become someone like Paul Farmer one day.

4

In the year 2000, the United Nations International Fund for Economic Development asked the brilliant Iranian film director, Abbas Kiarostami, to travel to Uganda and make a film about the plight of orphans who had lost their parents due to AIDs and war. Kiarostami's *ABC Africa* emerged directly out of his ten-day trip to Uganda.[9]

In a densely populated urban neighborhood, children play before and *at* the cameras and cameramen busy at work. There is no colonizing or even humanitarian gaze here. The children almost frolic. There is a playful, gamboling quality to the film shooting and cutting, too. The cameraman sometimes seems to lose control, as unruly children disrupt his filming with ambivalence and charming, insistent play. The film has no voice-over; omniscient narration has no place here. Using hand-held digital and still cameras, the film insists—lyrically so—on the beautiful and ugly, the seen and the unseen. Kiarostami fills his film surfaces with orphans, adopting Ugandan women, and taxi drivers, with heads, "faces, clapping hands, and skin" in "movement, gestures, and intonations." The result is "an open social world—one in which Kiarostami himself joins" as he inserts himself with camera into grimy, colorful Kampala with city kids, dancing and chanting.[10]

Kiarostami's car drives through city streets and nearby countryside too, recording passing scenes. The award-winning filmmaker is known for creating "poetry in motion" in and through film. *ABC Africa's* poetry includes dark moments. There are AIDS clinic scenes amidst others about an NGO for orphans, organized by hard-working Ugandan women and AIDS widows, who commit themselves to raising a child for a ten-year period. At one point, the camera pans into a clinic for children dying of AIDS, and then follows as one dead child's body is wrapped up in a blanket. Then, the staff and kin join in placing this bundle into a makeshift coffin made from a large cardboard box. Finally, this package of death is mounted on the back of a bicycle and wheeled away.[11]

Another scene takes place in complete darkness; the screen is black as voices sound. Kiarostami and his cameraman are arriving back to their hotel late at night, after the electric power has been cut for the night. They speak together in Farsi while groping to find their rooms. "Imagine that grandmother living with 35 kids," begins one. Imagine living "half of their life in the dark," quips the other. "Humans can adapt to anything" is the reply.[12] The film *ABC Africa*, however, is less about adaptation than it is about privilege and inequality, the wrongheadedness of pity in the face of complex, caring lives and sometimes irrepressible, mischievous glee.

Most remarkable is the way Kiarostami *sutures* in scenes of a special, more anomalous adoption. Suturing is precisely the word I mean here. The Ugandan orphan is an infant girl, and the new parents who adopt her are an Austrian couple. We watch at one point as these surrogate parents explain their decision to adopt a child—this new daughter—from Africa. With restraint and a touch of self-satisfaction, they speak of removing her from a world of disease and squalor. Kiarostami cuts in—sutures—a few additional brief scenes of these new white European parents with their black orphan child. In the longest, their impeccably dressed daughter plays in a brand new T-shirt, displaying one of Africa's controversial AIDS slogans: ABC ("Abstinence, Be faithful, use a Condom"). This sanitized adoptee plays *solo* on the carpet of a safe, posh international hotel in Kampala, while the new parents dine at a distance. Whether this scene *depicts* uneasiness or not, it *produces* nervousness, at least among most spectators from the North. Identifying with the subtle, selfish desires of these adopting parents on the one hand, but exposed to the film's juxtapositions, which suggest humanitarian entitlement, social isolation, and a reduction of joy, viewers find themselves torn, disturbed. They can comprehend the couple's wish to rescue "a seeming unfortunate."[13] But the scenes of Kiarostami also show another kind of stranger, with cameras and from Iran, partaking in scenes of jubilant children who challenge the intruding cameras (and those wielding them) in their midst with play.

In sum, the film brilliantly upsets kneejerk spectator positions of horror and pity, the kind we have all known from turning on our televisions and watching the evening news, or opening the humanitarian appeals that arrive in our digital devices on a daily basis. The straighter, less informal shots of the adopting Austrian couple also work to force identification. After all, this could be you or me, trying to work out personal grief about childlessness or infertility through a global strategy.

We might say that Kiarostami's film is something like multi-sited ethnography in simultaneous film mode. Just as the Kampala NGO of strong Ugandan women is doing noble work, this couple from the global North is also there, securing a future for themselves. In these straighter, steadier shots, some with the Austrian couple, some with the Ugandan widows, there is no challenging of the cameras. Nor are the filmmakers visible—or audible. Missing, though obvious, is the work of international adoption agencies with their persuasive advertisements based on a global iconography of rescue—orphan rescue—a subject that feminist historian, Laura Briggs, has written about searingly.[14]

Kiarostami complicates Africa and humanitarianism, haunting spectators in the process. His sutured mix of scenes pushes viewers toward a more critical understanding about the jarring worlds that coexist—and sometimes collide—in Africa every day. In the final sequence, the couple and orphan daughter board a plane for Vienna. Is this solo Ugandan child a lucky girl? Kiarostami refuses to answer. His film closes in fictionalized, ironic mode with hyperbole instead: billowing cumulus clouds transform themselves into human faces, some still living beneath the sky in multiple, differentiated places. By avoiding the didactic and problematizing the humanitarian, Kiarostami did something remarkable: he subverted the movie's commissioning by a United Nations agency. Instead, he cut in the awkward and uncomfortable. Let's be clear: he sutured in you and me.

5

Suturing is not an easy concept—or practice. With these two examples of suturing at work—a patient's patched hospital bedding and an ironic filmmaker's take on orphan work in and out of Africa—may its implications for historians widen. Now, I turn to some of the challenges of cut-like editing that I have faced in assembling a new kind of African medical history.

A Nervous State: Violence, Remedies, and Reverie in Colonial Congo marries biopolitics with the securitization of power and health, a theme most fitting for our brave new world of global health. It joins these two aspects with vernacular public healing, that is, forms of therapeutic work and refusal by communities of African subjects.[15] It is a complex history with many subjects, positions, and narrative strands. It has taught me the importance of carefully *suturing in* refractory evidence, in part so that my readers not only learn about the past but think about our common present.

A key standard has been *not* to focus on biomedicine alone. Colonial medicine is there, but the book equally attends to the positive and negative registers—the healing *and* warlike qualities—of African therapeutics. *A Nervous State* is about biomedical research and health care in the Equateur region of the Belgian Congo, once King Leopold's notorious Congo Free State. In this humid region of equatorial forest, imperial conquest and forced extraction of wild-growing rubber combined. The results were shockingly violent and brutal. Most of my readers will know about cut-off human hands, the international human rights scandal, and *King Leopold's Ghost*.[16] What is less well known is how strongly the historical record suggests reproductive maladies became rife, during and after this early colonial period, when sex of various kinds—coerced, violent, commercialized, marital, and protection-seeking—produced an epidemic of gonorrhea and other STDs, quite likely chlamydia among them. A long decade of deadly sleeping sickness, mixed with war, hunger, and flight, produced high mortality and refugee rates in the 1900s. And, afterwards, a strongly biopolitical regime, the successor state (the Belgian Congo) placed a strong emphasis on demographic, gynecological, venereal, and infertility research from the 1920s on. Clinical surveys and research, injections and care played themselves out in relation to African populations alternately seen as frail, sickly, and "dying out" from "malaise" or "race suicide," or as feisty, vengeful, not yet subdued.

My history is about confrontation and conflict in the Equateur region between Congolese subjects and various categories of colonizing Europeans—state doctors, territorial administrators, company agents, traders, plantation owners, missionaries, nurses, and wives. *A Nervous State* elaborates five long moments or events when state power and vernacular healing came to loggerheads, from the 1900s through the 1950s. In the 1950s, the Belgian colonial state was busy constructing an infertility clinic in Equateur, not far from a special penal colony built to contain and punish therapeutic, religious rebels. From the 1930s, these struggles involved state force and state persons acting in two different guises of power: a nervous, security-oriented guise and a biopolitical one. The latter was oriented toward promoting life and health; the first aimed at arresting and containing public healing, sorcery-laced rumors, and therapeutic forms of rebellion.

The shift I am making may be subtle but it does reinvent the range that a medical historian of Africa must cover. Rather than trying to convince my readers that African therapeutics was a parallel way of knowing illness and practicing health care, I trace how colonial dichotomous thinking, which pitted Western science against vernacular "superstition," worked as politics with technologies and over time in a specific situation. My heuristic of a two-faced state gives me not a dichotomy nor two parallel worlds, but a triangular formulation: the state directed towards suffering, health, and fecundity on the one hand, *and* the state directed at security problems, on the other. Indeed, Africans used medicines in war and in healing, and their use of terror medicines in battle were a significant issue from the time Henry Morton Stanley and others first blasted uncooperative villages with gunfire in the nineteenth century.

6

Why do I find the word suturing helpful in this work? The Belgian Congo state operated in the face of Congolese forest populations; profoundly violated (sometimes losing hands or feet), they remained fretful about survival, fertility, pregnancy, and social reproduction. These persons, who had memories of dreadful rubber wars and devastation in their beings, had long used dance, song, landscape, and medicines to purge the toxic and mend their bodies and worlds. If healing and harming is a common pair in sub-Saharan Africa, as Steven Feierman has long suggested,[17] in these parts of central Africa, the more salient social and bodily pair is about purging and reweaving, eliminating and mending.[18]

My treatment situates Congo's iconic imperial violence of the 1890s and 1900s in a decidedly non-epic history, which suggests that this past should not be disconnected from Congo's recent, ongoing, post-1996 time of war and rape in the Democratic Republic of Congo. There are no heroes or villains in my history, though there is massacre and mutilation. Rather, my subject is the event and structure of violence, its duration and reproduction across generations, through bodies, imaginations, and intellects. This historical process, which entailed somatic processes across time and generations, was mediated through colonial medical research and through African public healing.

The notion of a colonial state with two relevant faces is my heuristic, and it opens up much. The nervous and biopolitical states became like parallel agencies, and they sharpened different, linked technologies. The first focused on security, crime, and fearful healing movements, the second on medicine, demography, and public health. The state was not abstract or homogeneous; highly bureaucratic and made up of persons, it—and they—fed on and fueled emotional states. The state's two faces often became like moods—one more guilty and humanitarian, the other nervous and energized by dread.

Combining medical and demographic technologies with penal techniques in the same history, and directing sustained attention to vernacular speech, practice, and imaging all the while, is a new way of framing an unfolding situation where, as Frantz Fanon told us now long ago, colonial medicine produced deep ambivalence.[19]

A fairly straightforward, chronological sweep of periods, events, and confrontations shapes the work. Within this trajectory and interrupting its sweep, however, I insert bits and layers of time, story, image, and memory to disorder and *snarl* a universal calendar of progressive time. Thinking about a patient's makeshift memory quilt of a hospital bed helps me here. But it is neither a patchwork nor domesticity that I am after in my suturing as historical composition. Rather, I usually work by clutching some fascinating bit, a perplexity of some kind, and then seek to suture it in somewhere, perhaps in a section devoted to event and story, perhaps in one more akin to structure and analysis. The surgical metaphor assists me: after all, a surgeon's seam-like joints and stitches tackle wounds and enable scars. And, my history of colonial Congo's Equateur must grapple, more than most African medical histories, with injuries and disfigurements, with evidentiary traces of colonial violence, memory, and forgetting of all kinds.[20] Prominent in my history are Equateur-born and Equateur-residing Congolese of all kinds: trappers, hunters, and fisherwomen; chiefs, clerks, porters, and taxpayers; dancers, cannabis growers, copal gatherers, and healers; catechists, mothers, and nurses; and from the 1950s, chauffeurs and urbane, strolling modern music stars. These subaltern and middle subjects made use of charms, dance, and song, as they sought decent lives, gaiety, bounty, and fame, and sometimes healing and revenge, too.

I share two examples of my work of suturing in historical writing here. The first involves splicing in some of my bursting material on Congolese imaginations and bodily practice. At my disposal is a rich vernacular archive of "oral tradition," most of it collected and assembled by some earnest, persistent Flemish missionary priests. If at first this poetic archive seemed to have a timeless, repetitive, difficult-to-date quality, over time I began to comprehend how it surfaced in and as event. Indeed, all the confrontations that I privilege *as event* involved the use of medicines, poisons, charms, rumors, and song, wielded by fed up persons and groups, often suffering and ill besides. The second example is about where to cut in one photograph so it jars.

7

Ewewe began as song in my evidence, a song about a mythological—perhaps once part historical—figure named Ewewe, whose grandson and granddaughter, Lianja and Nsongo, used to come to life often in performance around village fires. A key Ewewe song goes like this:

> Ewewe, kiii
> Ewewe, kiii
> We show out Ewewe
> Ewewe, we escort you away

Ki, ki, ki
Give us food,
Give us fish
Ewewe kiii
We are going to usher out Ewewe,
Nsongo and Lianja, kiii
Sweep away sickness,
Carry away coughs
Ewewe, kiii
Give us food.[21]

Ewewe was much more than its lyrics alone. Ewewe was a festive drama periodically performed to eliminate illness and affliction, provide and receive food, and weave together health among contiguous villages in a common effort of purging and mending. Negative, harmful energy, matter, even persons or corpses could also be eliminated in the process, to link, relink, and weave back together anew through Ewewe's wrapped up corpse as a bundle of energy and debris: such was the healing, recycling process. Ewewe would be carried up high through villages until the package of death yielding life, the container enclosing his spirit and force, reached the big river, where the porter figures placed the Ewewe bundle in the river. It floated away. (Something not dissimilar is glimpsed in the *ABC Africa* film: kin push a wrapped package of a corpse away from the AIDS clinic by bicycle, toward funeral rituals that will reconnect kin and neighbors with spirits in therapeutic, festive ways, connecting the living with the dead and easing loss and grief in the process).

Closely related persons living in the Equateur zone—who sometimes called themselves Mongo, Nkundo, Elinga, and Ekonda—performed Ewewe in the 1920s, 1930s, 1940s, likely for most of the 19th century, probably much earlier too. A Flemish missionary described an Ewewe performance as an epidemic removal procession.[22] The music of this structured, patterned dance sometimes became the whistles and pounding footsteps of its porter men alone. These men and youth were busy carrying the corpse of the grandfather of the central mythological figure in these people's ironic moral imaginations: a hunter, trapper, magician of a figure known as Lianja. An Ewewe procession produced nervousness while it escorted Ewewe from one village to the next with special transitional work as one set of porters passed his covered dead body on to the next group of carriers. As performance, Ewewe worked by producing fear and joy, wonder and daydreams. It removed the rotting waste and cadaverous body of this ancestral figure whose grandson, Lianja, has been a favorite epic hero of Africanist folklorists for generations. Africa's oral tradition specialists have tended to treat the Lianja epic as a text or as a recreational performance, however, rather than as integral to vernacular practice about reproducing worlds through elimination and renewal.

Coupled with this social logic were concerns about bodily flow. Therapeutic ritual embraced enema logic and practice, moving medicines into and debris out of an ailing person's body. This form of regional public healing and intimate hygiene, therefore, is much more than vernacular *color* within my historical writing. Ewewe and associated phenomena are more like a critical, energizing force within historical process and event.

8

Consider Kiarostami's *ABC Africa* once again. Historical writing may entail parallel kinds of suturing in awkward clips, including material about some of the self-serving, self-justifying persons who parachuted into colonial life as doctors, magistrates, territorial administrators, traders, and missionaries. Colonial mobility was less about quick arrivals for errands and consultancies, however; it involved longer, deeper entanglements in African situations, clinics, and missions. But humanitarian impulses combined with personal strategies of reproduction nonetheless.

As a historian, I tend to be less elliptical than Kiarostami when I tackle sources revealing the goals, fantasies, and self-deceit of my subjects. My characters include a provincial doctor who arrived on the scene as a colonial technician at the height of 1930s hysteria over a low birth rate. As Dr. Schwers became the doctor in charge, he received orders and funding to do a large medical survey in 1936. The idea was to analyze the determinants of childless villages and the excess of deaths over births, and this across the same wide region that had known a brutalizing rubber economy of raiding, plunder, and death in the 1890s and 1900s.

Today, with anthropologists busy investigating science and experimentality in Africa's present,[23] this history of experimental biomedicine in the face of "race suicide" is valuable. Schwers' research and reporting ultimately suggest incompetence, fed by career anxieties and extinction fantasies, and combined with a determined effacement of a deeply violent past. Still, scientific experimentality is not enough; we must also unearth how African therapeutics burst forth into visibility again and again.

At a time when biomedicine meant research much more than care, confrontations with the two prongs of the colonial state in Dr. Schwers' years were, in part, over forced gynecological exams. Congolese women were engrossed at the time in other kinds of vernacular practice that mixed public healing with dissent and refusal. The nervous state and the biopolitical state clashed with each other, *and* with missionaries in the area, *and* with these Congolese involved in practices of elimination. Ewewe-like gestures—sweeping out and purging, with song and dance in public, but also inside women's bodies—were part of the healing spectacles known as *likili*. Dancers used broom-like flywhisks to gesture their distaste and suggest a sweeping out of doctors intruding into their lives and bodies. As they did so, and then for years afterwards too, Dr. Schwers kept speaking of shock and endocrinology. Ultimately his language blamed the colonized for being frail, "degenerate," and unable to rally in the face of "civilization." Yet the fact that vernacular gynecological ritual intensified in this context complicates the history of this region where demographic sampling suggested that about one in three women were suffering from barrenness in the 1950s.

Scholars of central African vernacular healing have long pointed to psychic and religious dimensions. From an epidemiological perspective, however, purging bodily insides—wombs—that already knew infection may well have driven sterilizing disease deeper into women's bodies. This kind of somatization has not received the attention it deserves. It is time to wonder about the way bodily and psychic wounds (including rape in the 1890s and 1900s),[24] internal cleansing practices, *and* infection endured, reproducing themselves across generations.

9

Thus, my first example of suturing is about stitching in the awkward figure of Dr. Schwers in relation to vernacular bodily ritual as dissent and as somatic, biological possibility. My second is about another kind of joining important for new historical writing. Sometimes it may mean showing how past and present were joined in everyday lives and daydreams, and differentially so. Sometimes, it may mean showing how the past could suddenly rear its presence within everyday life or within a historical subject's diary, song, or in a funereal, festive dance performance.

Usually I seek to *suture in* when confronted with something unusual, startling, or uncanny in a primary source. When I first stumble upon this anomalous bit, my question to self instantly becomes: where in the world am I going to insert this nugget? How can I work it in *not* seamlessly perhaps, but so it sticks out, so it catches and *jars*. I seek less the suture that slowly dissolves from sight, therefore, but more to produce a crooked scar that forces wonder and disquiet.

A few years ago, I spent ten days in Nashville, Tennessee, working in the archives of the Disciples of Christ mission by day (and listening to live country music and the blues at night). Three mission doctors who worked in Congo's Equateur left behind papers and photographs of note. The first, Dr. Royal J. Dye grew up posing for photographs with his regal first name and a fancy bicycle in Ionia, Michigan. When Dr. Dye came back from Congo about 1902, he orchestrated photographs of himself as an imperial, tropical doctor star with exotic loot to display. He had been in Congo at the height of atrocious violence associated with the rubber boom and bust, but only his wife left behind traces about some of the violence of this time. The second doctor was an irascible hunter from Texas. Dr. Jaggard was easily irked whenever he sensed the pomposity of his doctor colleagues working in the large mission hospital near the provincial capital. A frontier man with a frontier mentality, Dr. Jaggard relished working in his remote bush hospital from where he could easily go out hunting, which he often did when fed up with the tedium of surgery and patient care. Research was the last thing ever on this missionary doctor's mind, but he left behind some compelling prose about the low birth rate. Dr. Jaggard stressed that forced labor in porterage work, malnutrition, and infection during childbirth were, together, making it difficult for women to conceive, conceive again, or carry pregnancies to term.

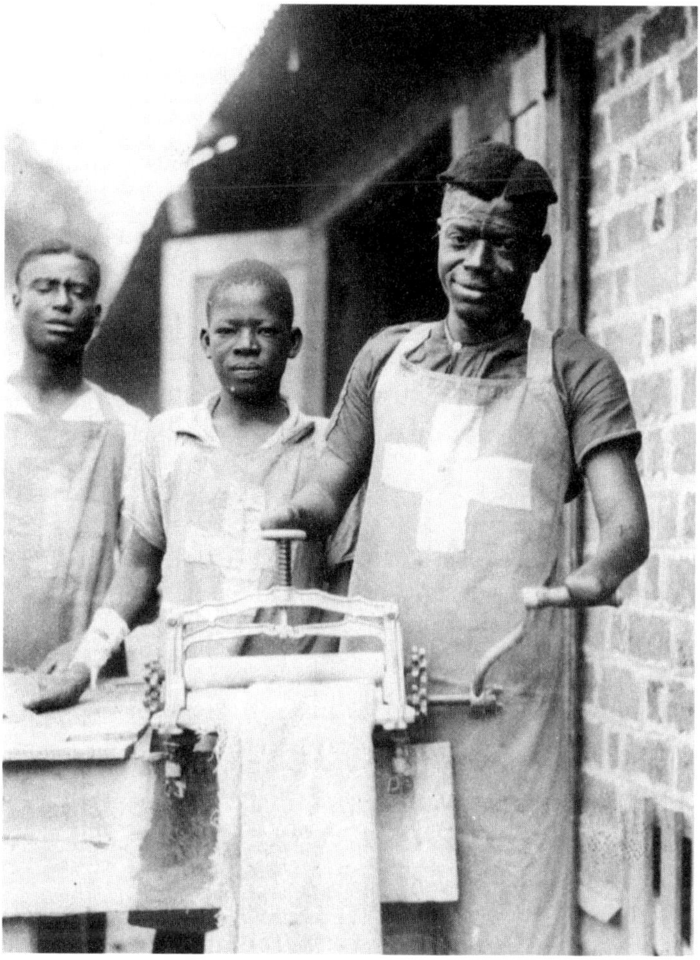

Bolenge Hospital medical assistant, ca. 1927 (courtesy of Disciples of Christ Historical Society, Nashville, Tennessee).

The third doctor was Dr. Barger; he was the interwar researcher of the three. He compiled a striking set of photographs about leprosy in adults and the treponemal disease, yaws (*pian* or *framboesie*) in children. I spent much of a day in Nashville moving from one Barger photograph to the next. Many were close-ups of leprosy and yaws. Some showed patients receiving injections or waiting on long benches outdoors. Others were staff photos, with Dr. Barger posing with his newly trained nurses and assistants. There were few close-ups among these, but there was one—a critically important one—of a hospital assistant whose job was to work the bandage pressing machine.

I gasped when I first saw this photograph from the 1920s. Most rubber violence had ended by 1906. I gasped, as iconic historical event and this man's intimate, autobiographical past suddenly, simultaneously parachuted themselves into my consciousness. Congolese with stumps for arms? Most of us know photographic images depicting them so, standing upright and posed in about 1904, wrapped in white cloth wrappers by a missionary photographer, their missing, cut-off hands gone, and their black arm ends displayed in high, white-black contrast for all to see. This kind of humanitarian photograph was ricocheting around the world in the early 20th century in magic lantern shows, where it served as ammunition in a propaganda war over conditions in King Leopold's Congo; and it has been in circulation ever since, especially in the last 15 years as journalists and humanitarian organizations have grappled with Congo's violent past and present and sought to stir emotions and donations through repeating exhibiting one of these shock-photos once again.

Dr. Barger's is the only photograph that seems to exist, however, that provides visual evidence about a victim who survived beyond this violent period of the "Rubber Wars," as the picture's verso explains. This hospital worker was adopted into everyday work life in this medical mission hospital at Bolenge in Congo's Equateur. The photograph speaks volumes to the way the past endured, and how it could suddenly turn up—visually—in plain daylight as a reminder, jarring those who witnessed the sight of such a person mutilated long before.

Where and how should I suture this frightening image into my historical narrative? I am not interested in haunting for haunting's sake. Nor am I interested in a spectral frame. My goal is not to shock today's readers as magic lantern shows did way back in the time of Roger Casement, E. D. Morel, and the evangelical, humanitarian campaign against atrocities in King Leopold's Congo.[25] But this photograph was never part of any magic lantern show. It tells us that visual, human reminders of a horrifically violent past, of disabling injury, were part of everyday life for those living in Equateur in the 1920s and 1930s, including the main doctor fantasizing extinction, Dr. Schwers. Indeed, it is beside this doctor's repetitious words and intrusive acts that this photograph belongs as a counterpoint sutured in.

Where are the biopolitics, humanitarianism, and security in all of this? They reside in this man's story and in the photograph of him. His traumatic injury occurred during war, at a time when removing hands from corpses and sometimes even live bodies became some combination of weapon, ritual, and bureaucratic routine. It was a time of intense nervousness everywhere, a colonial state terrified and struggling, while the Bolenge mission huddled, quietly working to rescue a few victims perhaps, but too nervous to lose their evangelical perch in Congo to raise much of a voice. Medicine was always part of their perch, and Dr. Dye got the hospital going as an evangelical humanitarian project of sorts in this same period. By the interwar period, Dr. Schwers was speaking about shock and extinction as if none of this violence had ever happened or might be related to reproductive disruption in the region. But Dr. Barger's photograph tells us that no one was allowed to forget so easily: not those living and working in Equateur, not even Dr. Schwers.

10

It is time to conclude. May these few reflections about suturing—in hospital home-making, in film-making, and in writing new medical histories for our 21st century present—go some way toward providing a sense of the urgencies and possibilities facing today's historians of medicine in Africa and beyond.

We have entered a significantly new era of producing medical histories of and for Africa. The shifts lie in economies and technologies; they involve intellectual shifts, neoliberalism, and new media. We can debate when this new era began and how to label it. But as the Basel conference program that inspired this essay demonstrates,[26] there is a fresh intensity of interest in unpacking the history of biomedical and global health research and care in Africa. What's going on, on the ground in Africa and globally, makes it new: we live in a tough, neoliberal world of structural violence, stark inequalities, unkempt wars, and biosecurity.

There are deep roots to biopolitical and security states, and these have involved profound entanglements with vernacular politics and the public healing of angry, suffering multitudes. The biopolitical-security nexus has not gone away, and it is here to stay. It is this nexus in our post-9/11 world of staggeringly risky disparities that is reproducing global health as a new realm of research, practice, industry, and higher education. It is urgent to know about—and historicize—how humanitarianism and securitization connect and combine. There is simply no way to do a historical ethnography of a Congo rape hospital today, for example, to examine how global health agendas are arriving there and being remade, without grappling with how the "I want to help" global health humanitarians are trying to transform lives and make careers out of this dire situation. Some are doing rounds of "clinical tourism;"[27] some keep their distance and consume information from websites about women at risk of rape in war. But major struggles for security—ongoing war—are driving an epidemic of sexualized violence while opening up this new global mental health frontier, where trauma technologies meet gynecology and feminist politics in strange keys.

The big point about suturing is as simple as this: *practice matters*. How we assemble our histories—what bits, persons, locations, and objects we select and combine—matters. We necessarily stitch as we go, so why not work even harder and seek to suture together incongruous, paradoxical, jarring bits of evidence? There is room to be more self-conscious about how we ask our readers to identify—and dis-identify—and with what and whom. We can theorize all we like, and we do need concepts and also to work with them in relation to empirical thens and theres, but our challenges lie in practice, in how we design our research, how we write or otherwise produce histories that embrace viewpoints, experiences, images, sounds, and a range of scales. This means taking multi-sitedness in more complex directions—well beyond metropole and colony, and well beyond Geneva, Atlanta, and some African postcolonial location somewhere, too. It means combining comparability with differential points of view.

Still, and no matter what, findings must be assembled into some kind of package. It is worth wondering long and hard about the fact that research need not result in a two-dimensional text any more. If books and bookstores are disappearing from our world—and the view from Ann Arbor, Michigan, where the global corporate headquarters of Borders bookstores recently closed their doors, suggests this is the case—the implications are many. At the same time, new digital, media, and communication technologies suggest not just transformed clinical worlds in Africa, with every medical worker and patient clutching a cell phone as they navigate illness. These new capacities suggest we need to think about producing more interactive products, especially since these may draw in and instruct larger and more complexly positioned audiences. Medical historians should be in the forefront of using new media to produce histories. Why? For one, because we have huge, eager audiences, some hungry for and others desperately needing more complex forms of understanding. We are also well positioned to access scientific, medical, and heritage monies to do our work.

Attention to audiences is key. How we position readers, viewers, and listeners matters. Call it spectator positioning, if you like. Regardless, we live in a world more saturated with images than ever before. If many images are used to shock, they are also open to various kinds of circulation and careful, thoughtful forms of suturing. The aesthetic level of suturing as craft—producing histories that are marvelous to read—is all fine and good. But the big thing that suturing as a concept gives us is a renewed awareness of audiences and thus of our capacity to strategically force learning and enable consciousness as we engage and disarm.

Everywhere I go, it seems, I am meeting middle class parents complaining about disconnected teenage children with their minds and fingers caught up in video games. I meet roughly the same age group in my undergraduate classes in Michigan: they are bright, and they are wired. They may not be keen to speak to their parents, but these video gamers are key players in our global world's ever growing "I want to help and rescue crowd." I am not (quite) suggesting that historians begin making video games, but some interactive global health teaching modules, grounded in concepts coming out of the best work in colonial medical histories, might do important work in steering the aspirations of this new generation of students beyond easy platitudes. Just imagine if every global health student and intern (from the North) received a strong dose of Frantz Fanon on colonial medicine and patient ambivalence[28] before landing in a clinic or refugee camp in Africa? I may be dreaming, but there is no gainsaying that the historical shallowness (if not obtuseness) of the global health and humanitarian fields would benefit from more historical knowledge, some of it sutured in as disturbing bits about the vexed historical positions of expatriate doctors, technicians, and helpers from the North.

Suturing means, in part, making links between pasts, presents, and positions in ways that jar and jolt. Thinking more about who our audiences are and who they might be requires thinking beyond our conventional spaces and objects of scholarly production. If more medical histories produced in Africa by those based in African history departments is a pressing agenda, so, too, are the challenges of preserving evidence: how to co-preserve and co-constitute medical archives and manuscripts. New media technologies allow for expanding production and preservation. With today's world a scary, teetering world of global health and dangerous inequities, and with Africa a continent where war zones and heritage monies go together with emerging medical markets and new kinds of digital devices, is it not time for a new era of creativity and suturing across registers and scales? Those earnest, eager students from the North, keen to travel and rescue must be kept in mind, as they are surely the global health workers, makers, and funders of the future. But they hardly should be our only public either. As new digital capacities transform how history is produced everywhere, may suturing be a concept that helps us think harder about how to sometimes unnerve while steadily broadening publics for medical history and the unfolding of global health in Africa.

ENDNOTES

1 Major research in ethnographic medical history in this same hospital and region in 1989–90 led to Nancy Rose Hunt, *A Colonial Lexicon: Of Birth Ritual, Medicalization, and Mobility in the Congo* (Durham: Duke University Press, 1999). On photography during my first trip back to the same region in 2007, see Nancy Rose Hunt, "Pharmacy Shops and Visual Culture in Kabila's Congo," *Alliances* (University of Michigan African Studies Center), no. 4 (Winter 2012): 10–11.

2 This original group included Steven Feierman, John Janzen, Gwyn Prins, and Murray Last, with two special issues in medical anthropology in *Social Science and Medicine* in 1979 (13, no. 4, edited by Janzen and Feierman) and 1981 (15, no. 3, edited by Janzen and Prins), and then in Steven Feierman and John Janzen, eds., *The Social Basis of Health and Healing in Africa* (Berkeley: University of California Press, 1992).

3 Tracy Kidder, *Mountains beyond Mountains: The Quest of Dr. Paul Farmer, a Man who would Cure the World* (New York: Random House, 2003). On the emergence of global health, see Craig R. Janes and Kitty K. Corbett, "Anthropology and Global Health," *Annual Review of Anthropology* 38 (2009): 167–83. That security has much to do with it is clear; see Stefan Elbe, *Security and Global Health: Towards the Medicalization of Insecurity* (Cambridge: Polity Press, 2010); Andrew Lakoff, *Biosecurity Interventions: Global Health and Security in Question* (New York: Columbia University Press, 2008). Global health is also a major new realm of biocapital; see Kaushik Sunder Rajan, *Biocapital: The Constitution of Postgenomic Life* (Durham: Duke University Press, 2006); and Aihwa Ong, "Scales of Exception: Experiments with Knowledge and Sheer Life in Tropical Southeast Asia," *Singapore Journal of Tropical Geography* 29 (2008): 117–29.

4 These definitions for "suture" follow closely those in the *Oxford English Dictionary (OED);* http://www.oed.com/. Second edition, 1989; online version March 2011.

5 Again, I closely follow the definitions given in the *OED*; http://www.oed.com/.

6 Dipesh Chakrabarty, "History and the Politics of Recognition," in *Manifestos for Historians,* ed. Keith Jenkins, Alan Munslow, and Susan Gordon (London: Routledge, 2007).

7 A useful starting point for the ways historical writing has changed and

why is Chris Lorenz, "History and Theory," in *The Oxford History of Historical Writing. Volume 5: Historical Writing Since 1945,* ed. Axel Schneider and Daniel Woolf (Oxford: Oxford University Press, 2011), 13–35; on the arrival of the digital in historical production, see Daniel Cohen and Roy Rosenzweig, *Digital History: A Guide to Gathering, Preserving, and Presenting the Past on the Web* (Philadelphia: University of Pennsylvania Press, 2005).

8 Suturing in this sense is not included in the OED, though there are entries in other Oxford reference sources; see: Daniel Chandler and Rod Munday, *A Dictionary of Media and Communication* (Oxford: Oxford University Press, 2011); and Ian Buchanan, *A Dictionary of Critical Theory* (Oxford: Oxford University Press, 2010). Useful are Kaja Silverman, *The Subject of Semiotics* (New York: Oxford University Press, 1983); and Stephen Heath, "Notes on Suture," first published in *Screen* 18 (Winter 1978); http://www.lacan.com/symptom8_articles/heath8.html.

9 Abbas Kiarostami, "ABC Africa," originally released 24 October 2001 (France), released by New Yorker Films, 21 June 2005, 85 min.

10 This section benefited from several critical reviews of "ABC Africa," notably the eleven reviews posted on the IMDb website, found at: http://www.imdb.com/title/tt0281534/reviews, especially those by Howard Schumman, "A Personal and Poetic Film," 8 May 2006; and jcappy, "Under the Clouds," 9 February 2010. See, too, Hajnal Kiraly, "Abbas Kiarostami and a New Wave of Spectator," *Acta Univ. Sapientiae, Film and Media Studies* 3 (2010): 133–42.

11 Howard Schumman, "A Personal and Poetic Film," 8 May 2006, http://www.imdb.com/title/tt0281534/reviews.

12 jcappy, "Under the Clouds," 9 February 2010, http://www.imdb.com/title/tt0281534/reviews.

13 The quotation and ideas here come from: Keith Uhlich, "ABC Africa," *Slant Magazine,* 24 June 2005, http://www.slantmagazine.com/film/review/abc-africa/1586.

14 Laura Briggs, "Mother, Child, Race, Nation: The Visual Iconography of Rescue and the Politics of Transnational and Transracial Adoption," *Gender & History* 15 (2003): 179–200.

15 Nancy Rose Hunt, *A Nervous State: Violence, Remedies, and Reverie in Colonial Congo* (Durham: Duke University Press, forthcoming). This new medical history is set in Congo's Equateur.

16 Many will have read the important book of this title by Adam Hochschild, *King Leopold's Ghost: A Story of Greed, Terrorism, and Heroism in Colonial Africa* (Boston: Houghton Mifflin, 1998).

17 Steven Feierman, *The Shambaa Kingdom: A History* (Madison: University of Wisconsin Press, 1974); and Steven Feierman, *Peasant*

Intellectuals: Anthropology and History in Tanzania (Madison: University of Wisconsin Press, 1990).

18 Particularly clear on the weaving dimensions is Renaat Devisch, *Weaving the Threads of Life: The Khita Gyn-Eco-Logical Healing Cult among the Yaka* (Chicago: University of Chicago Press, 1993).

19 Frantz Fanon, "Medicine and Colonialism," in *A Dying Colonialism* (New York: Grove Press, 1994), 121–46.

20 See Nancy Rose Hunt, "An Acoustic Register, Tenacious Images, and Congolese Scenes of Rape and Ruination," in Special Issue on "Imperial Debris," ed. Ann Laura Stoler, *Cultural Anthropology* 23 (2008): 220–53.

21 E. Boelaert, "La procession de Lianja," *Aequatoria* 25, no. 1 (1962): 1–9, esp. 2.

22 Ibid.

23 Vinh-Kim Nguyen, "Government-by-exception: Enrolment and Experimentality in Mass HIV Treatment Programmes in Africa," *Social Theory & Health* 7 (2009): 196–217; Richard Rottenburg, "Social and Public Experiments and New Figurations of Science and Politics in Postcolonial Africa," *Postcolonial Studies* 12 (2009): 423–40; and P. Wenzel Geissler and Catherine Molyneux, eds., *Evidence, Ethos and Experiment: The Anthropology and History of Medical Research in Africa* (Oxford: Berghahn Books, 2011).

24 Hunt, "An Acoustic Register."

25 A point I make forcefully in Hunt, "An Acoustic Register."

26 "The History of Health Care in Africa: Actors, Experiences, and Perspectives in the 20th Century," conference at the University of Basel, 12–14 September 2011.

27 The expression is Claire Wendland's; see her "Moral Maps and Medical Imaginaries: Clinical Tourism at Malawi's College of Medicine," *American Anthropologist* 114 (2012): 107–21.

28 Fanon, "Medicine and Colonialism."

CARL SCHLETTWEIN LECTURES

The distinguished lecture of the Centre for African Studies Basel is held in remembrance of Dr. h.c. Carl Schlettwein, who played an important part in the development of African Studies at Basel and in the establishment of our Centre. His moral support was supplemented by the generous and farsighted assistance he gave to these activities. Carl Schlettwein was born in Mecklenburg in 1925 and emigrated to South Africa in 1952. Until 1963 he lived in South West Africa, the former German colony that was then under South African administration. When he married Daniela Gsell he moved to Basel. In 1971 Schlettwein founded the Basler Afrika Bibliographien (BAB) as a library and publishing house in order to allow international institutions to access bibliographic information on South West Africa (Namibia). Accordingly, he published the first national bibliography on this African country. Through these activities the BAB contributed to documenting and researching a nation with a particularly difficult history. Other publications dealt with historical, literary and geo-methodological topics, and included titles on Swiss-African relations. From an individualistic private initiative, the BAB developed into an institution open to the public and became a cornerstone of the Centre for African Studies Basel. As the Namibia Resource Centre – Southern Africa Library the institution is of world-wide importance. The Carl Schlettwein Stiftung, which was founded in 1994, runs the BAB and supports students and projects in Namibia as well as in other southern African countries. At present it funds the chair for African History with a focus on southern Africa in the Department of History of the University of Basel, as well as a lectureship in Southern African literature. The University of Basel honoured Carl Schlettwein with an honorary doctorate in 1997.

Carl Schlettwein Lectures

edited by the Centre for African Studies Basel

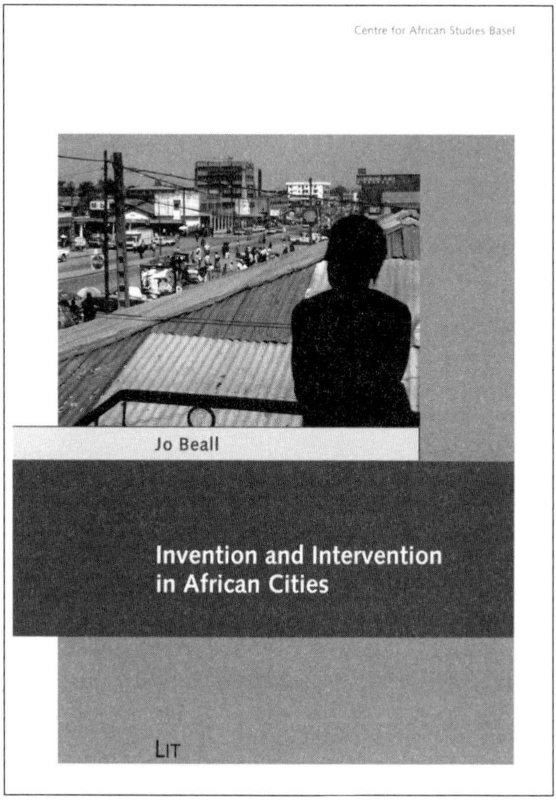

Jo Beall
Invention and Intervention in African Cities
Urban growth in Africa is higher than anywhere but, unlike earlier urbanisation trends in the industrialised world, it is not being accompanied by economic growth. The result is a continent that boasts high levels of poverty and inequality and the highest proportion of urban slum dwellers anywhere. Yet Africa has the least developed institutional architecture and infrastructure at the urban scale to effectively respond and to put in place the appropriate policy, regulatory and fiscal environment to address the social challenges of rapid urbanisation.
vol. 6, 2011, 56 pp., 9,90 €, br., ISBN-CH 978-3-643-80106-7

LIT Verlag Berlin – Münster – Wien – Zürich – London
Auslieferung Deutschland / Österreich / Schweiz: siehe Impressumsseite

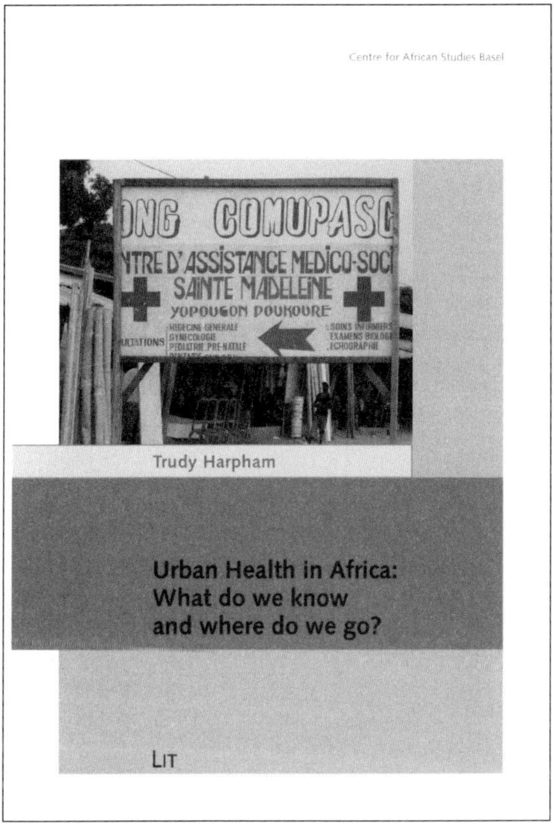

Trudy Harpham
Urban Health in Africa
What do we know and where do we go?

We have a certain amount of knowledge of the problems of urban health in Africa. We also partly understand the determinants of such problems: environmental, social, structural, and service related. Multi-level research has enabled the role of 'place' for health to be acknowledged and in particular, the importance of social connections at the neighbourhood level. However, truly multi-sectoral action for urban health, which reflects the multiple determinants, is rare and often fails. Pilot projects are rarely scaled up. More evaluative intervention research is needed and researchers need to engage policy makers at earlier stages. We also need to understand the urban policy process more - especially the role of frontline workers in determining policy.

Urban health research has focussed on problems (vulnerabilities) and not strengths or resilience. Using a more positive model of urban health might enhance the research translation process (getting research into policy and practice: GRIPP) and speed up action to improve urban health.

vol. 5, 2010, 56 pp., 9,90 €, br., ISBN-CH 978-3-643-80053-4

LIT Verlag Berlin – Münster – Wien – Zürich – London

Auslieferung Deutschland / Österreich / Schweiz: siehe Impressumsseite